About Ryah Summer-Cree and Mindful Momma-Affirmations and Coloring Pages to Manifest the Birth You Desire

LunaRose Create was started in 2022 by Ryah Summer-Cree. Inspired by the two very different births she'd experienced (a non-medically necessary c-section and hbac home birth after cesarean) this project of love was created. What was once an idea has turned into a collection of work and a small business. Her debut work Mindful Momma centers around the journey of pregnancy, birth, and motherhood. It was developed to instill confidence, autonomy, peace, and reassurance in all mothers regardless of where or how they birth their baby. Ryah Summer-Cree and LunaRose Create develops content that empowers and uplifts women.

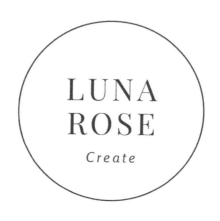

LUNA
ROSE

Create

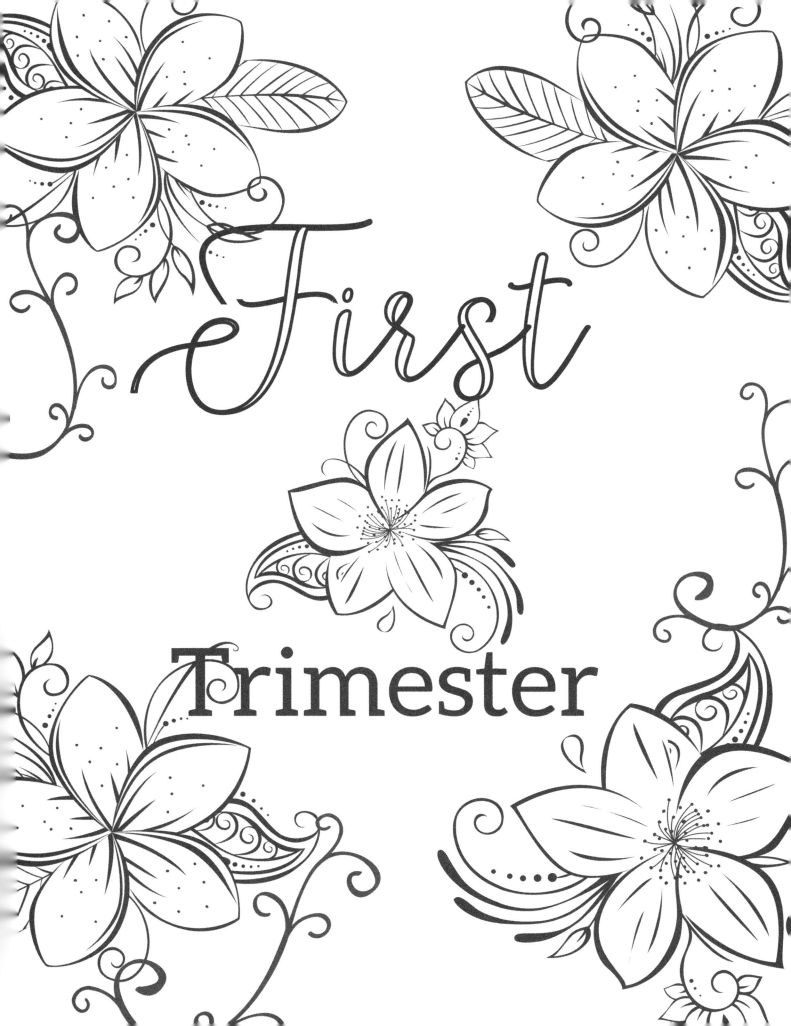

First
Trimester

I embrace and acknowledge

ALL THE EMOTIONS I'M FEELING. I WELCOME THIS NEW JOURNEY.

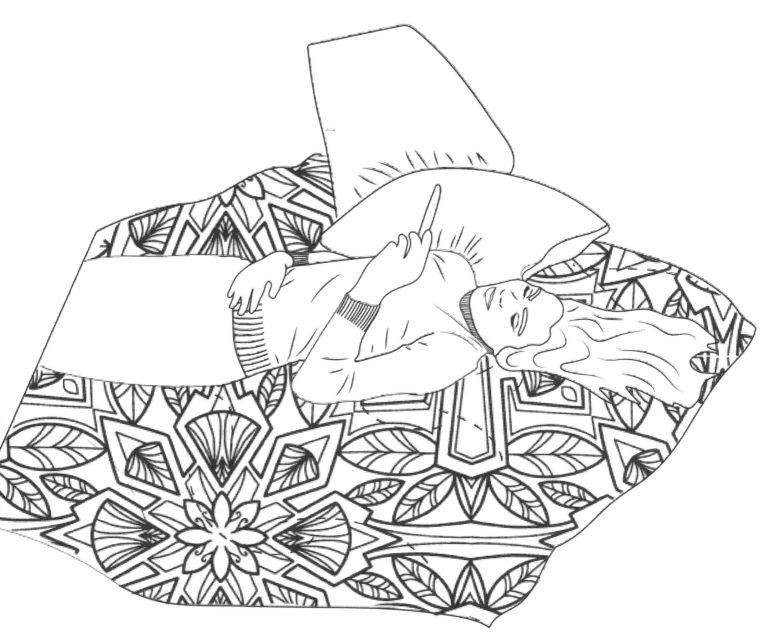

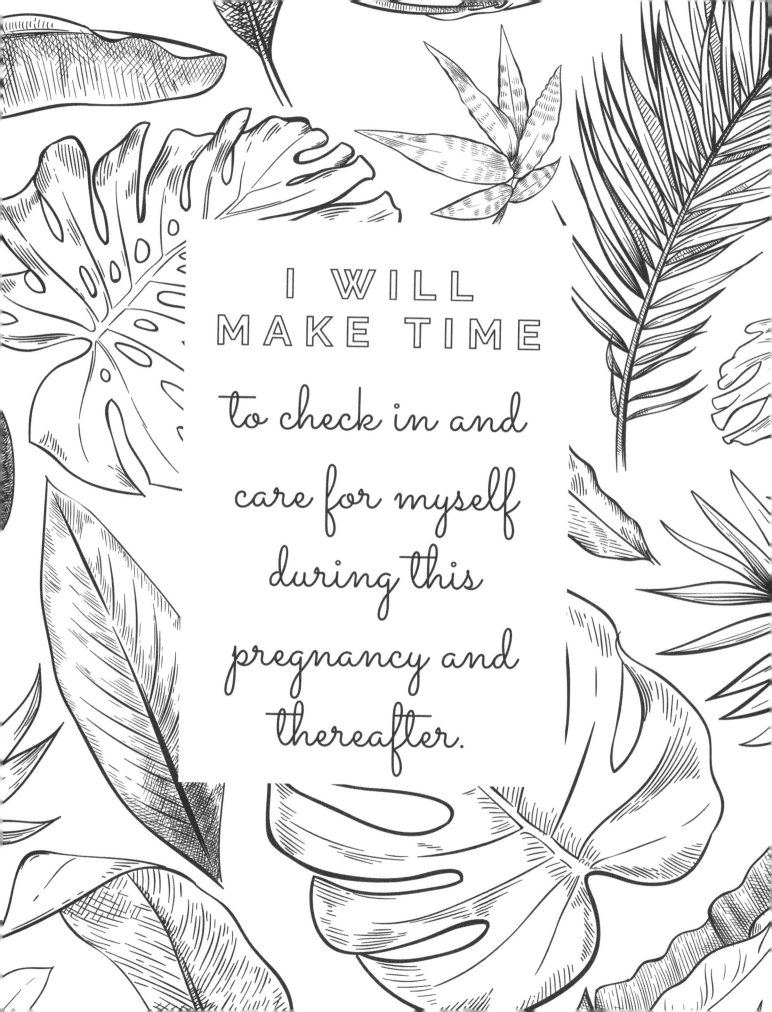

I WILL MAKE TIME to check in and care for myself during this pregnancy and thereafter.

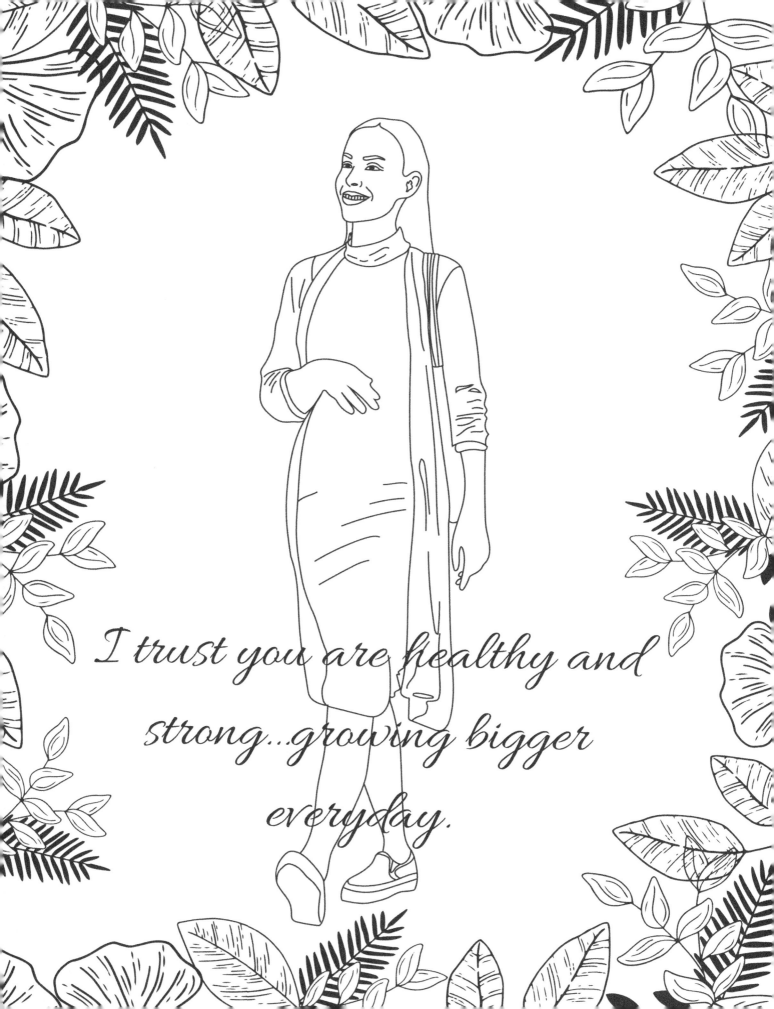

I trust you are healthy and strong...growing bigger everyday.

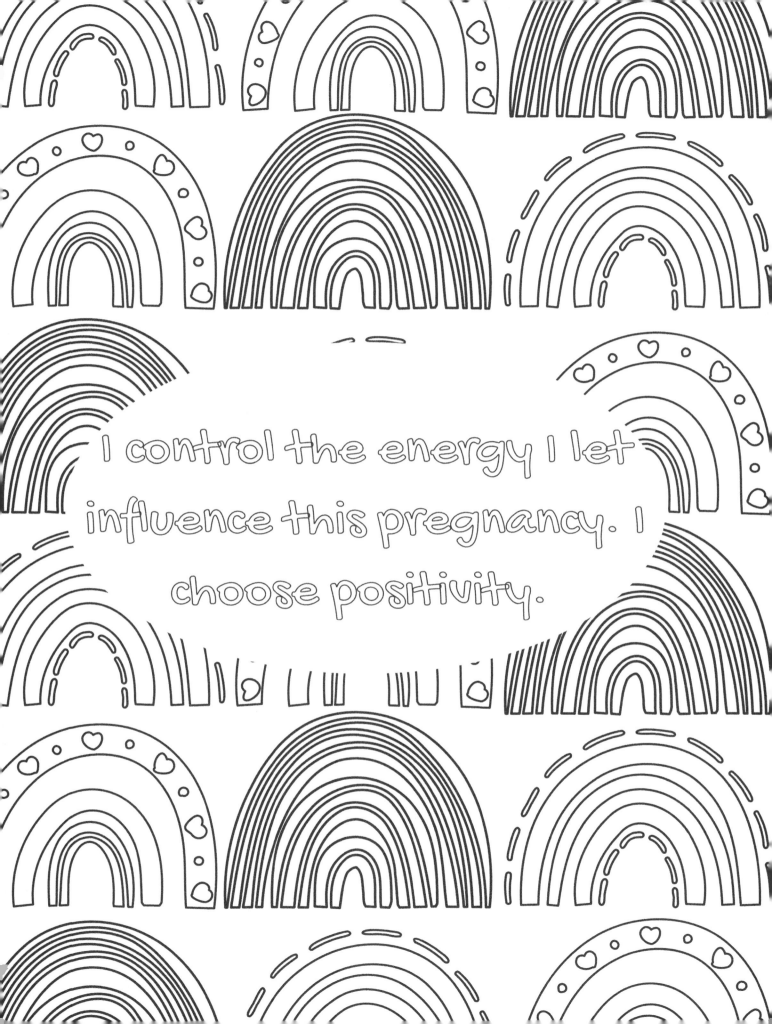

I control the energy I let influence this pregnancy. I choose positivity.

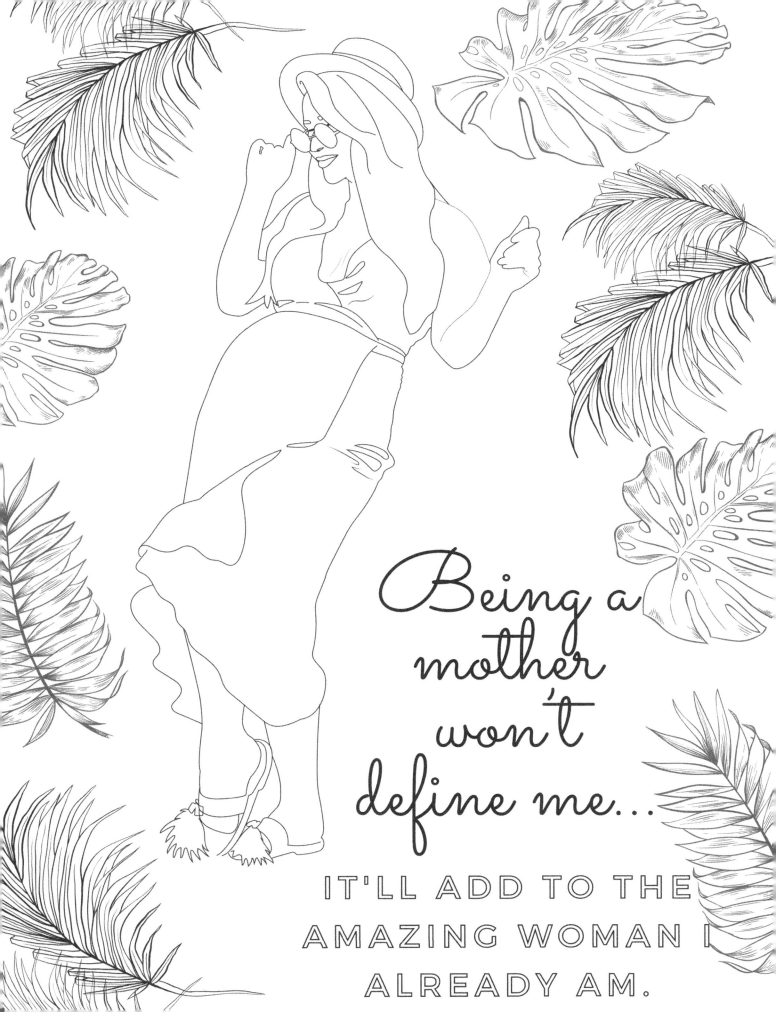

Being a mother won't define me...

IT'LL ADD TO THE AMAZING WOMAN I ALREADY AM.

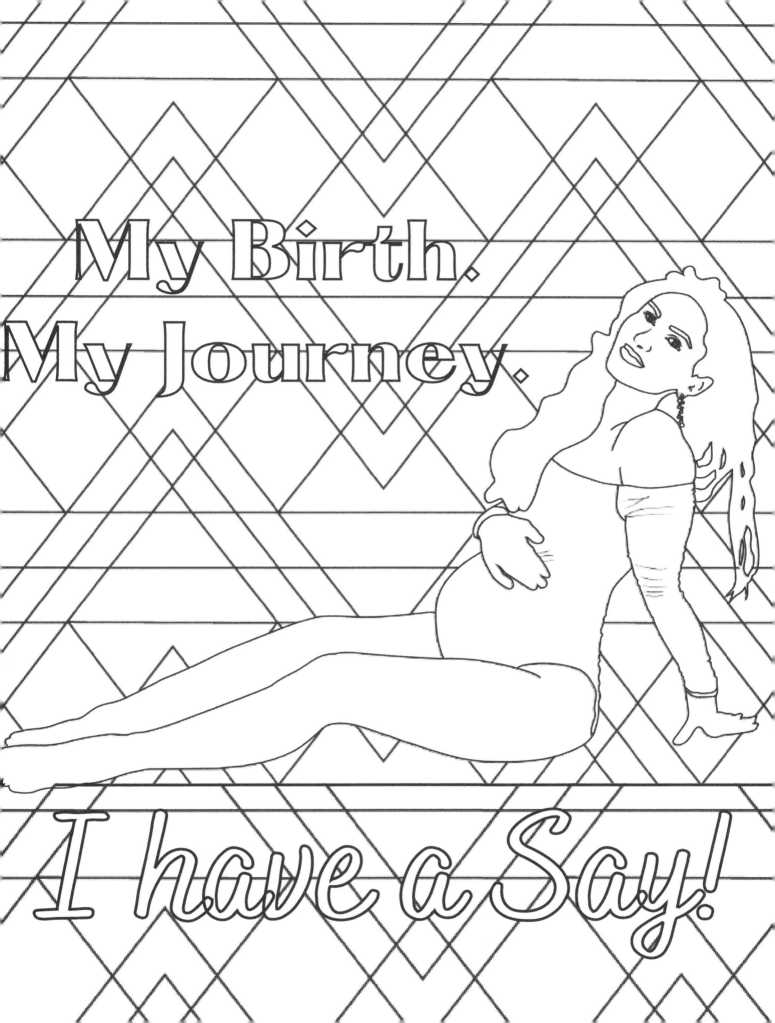

I enjoy educating myself on pregnancy and birth, and gain confidence in my ability to make the best choices for my baby and me.

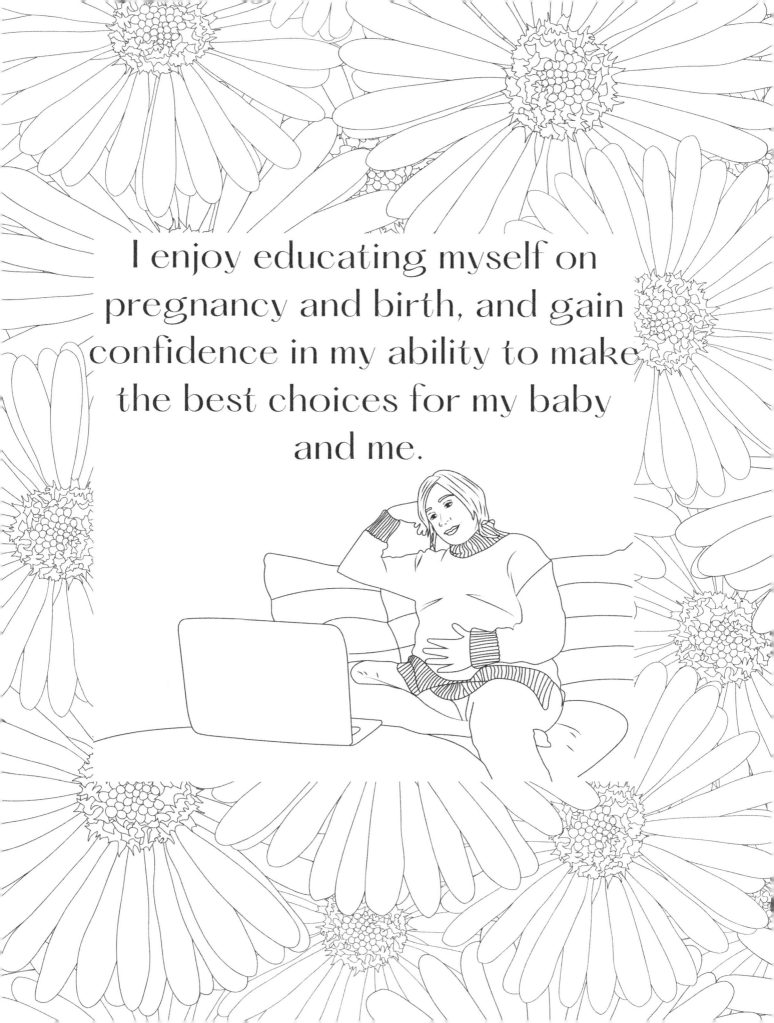

I've chosen the best team

TO SUPPORT ME IN LABOR AND AFTER

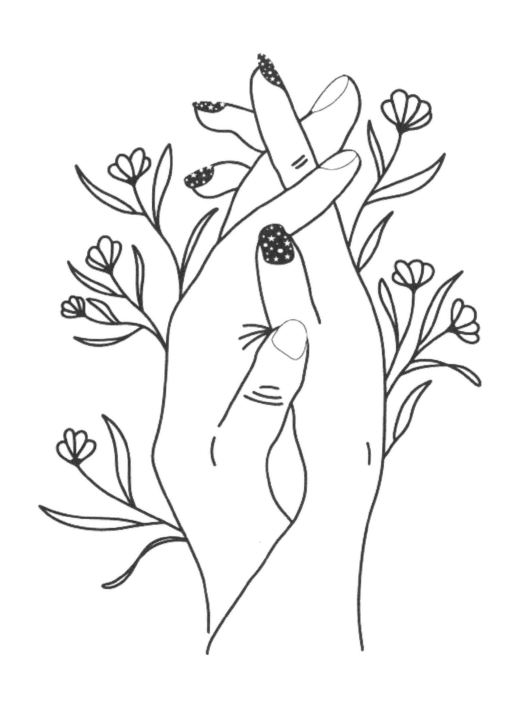

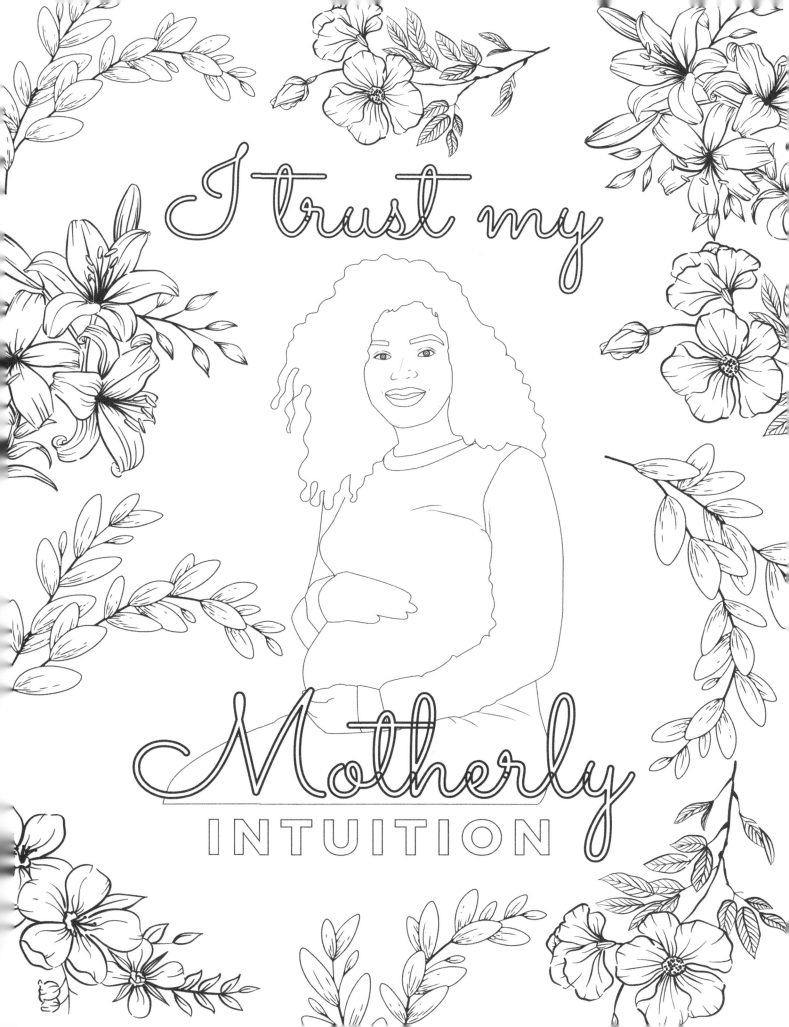

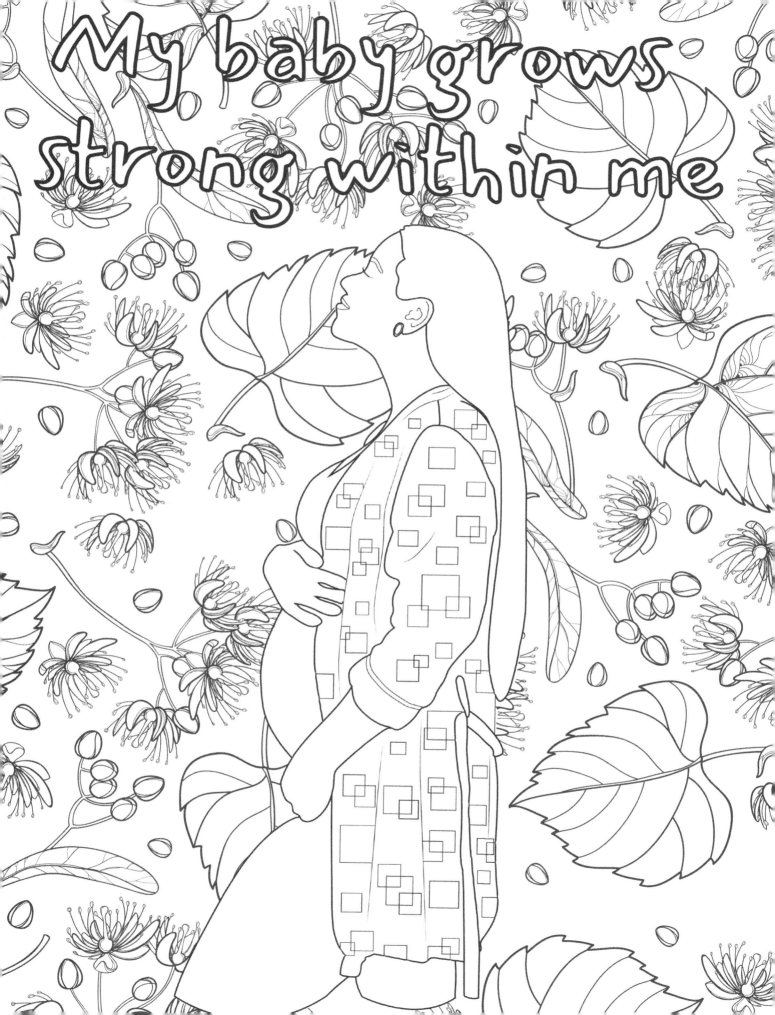

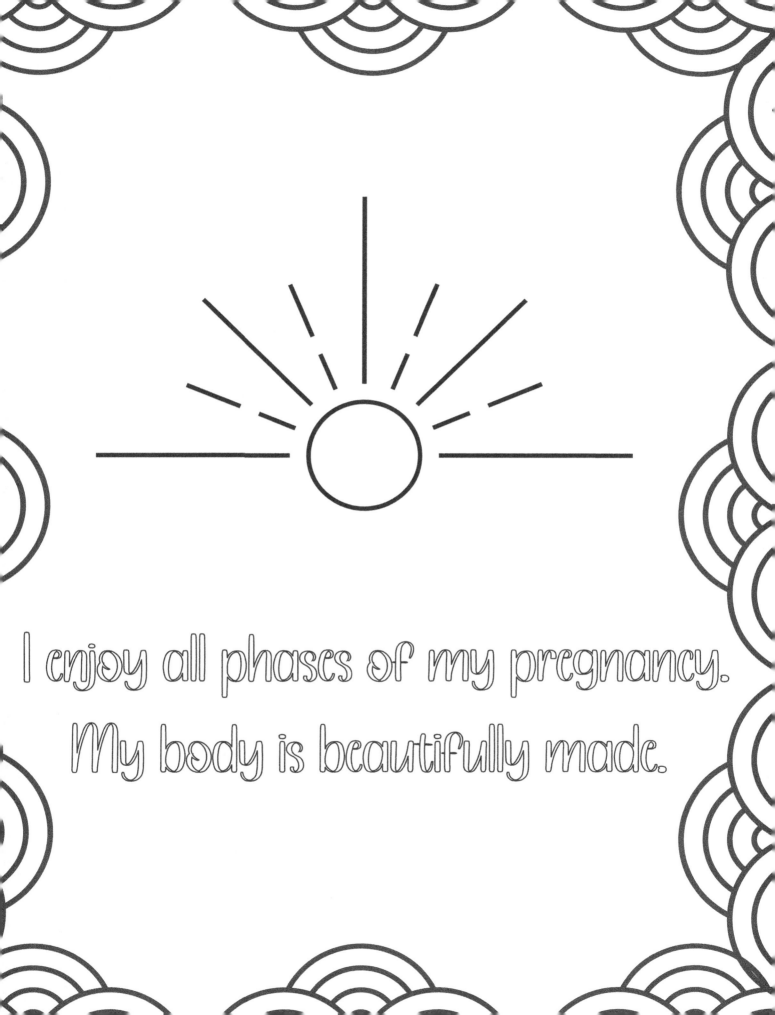

I enjoy all phases of my pregnancy.
My body is beautifully made.

No matter the gender of my baby we will form a

close and loving bond

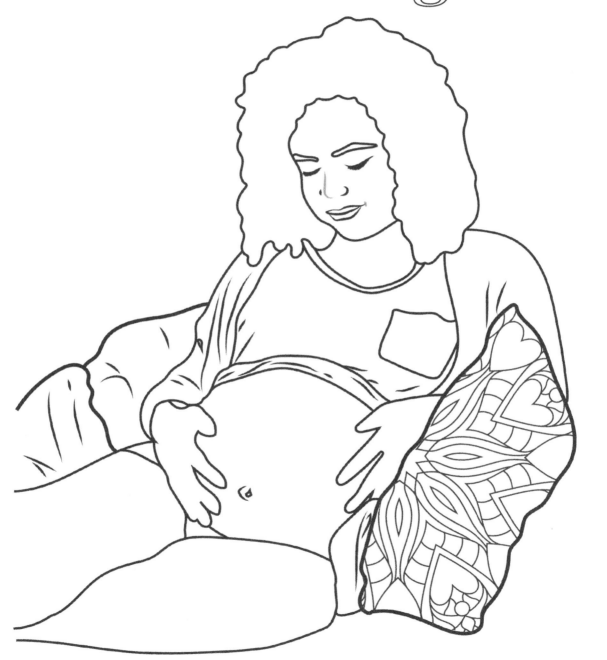

that will last a lifetime.

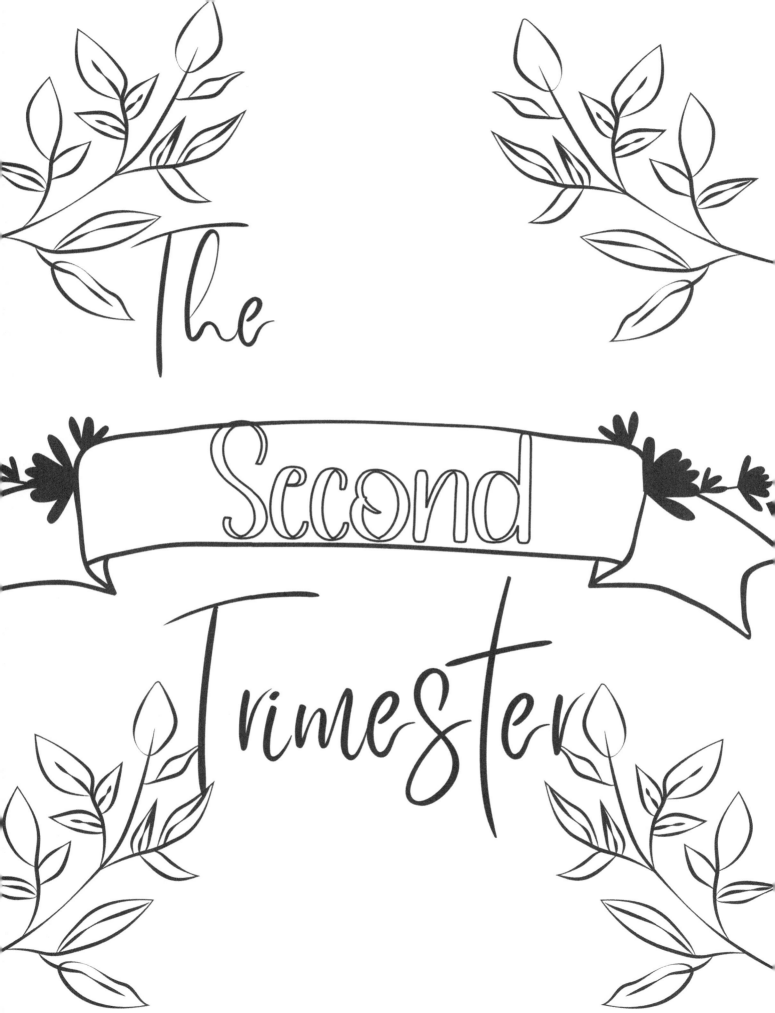

The Second Trimester

Releasing fear

Pregnancy and birthing your baby can often be met with uncertainty and fear. While it's important to acknowledge and educate yourself on all possibilities and outcomes, that doesn't mean you have to claim them.

Talk to your care provider, create a plan for the concerns you have, and then let those fears go. Focus on the pregnancy you want to have and the birth you've always wished for.

Believe that you are capable of having both. That you deserve both. When those fears creep in remind yourself that you've chosen the best team to support and care for you and your baby, that a plan has been made if anything should arise, and that you can do this....because you can.

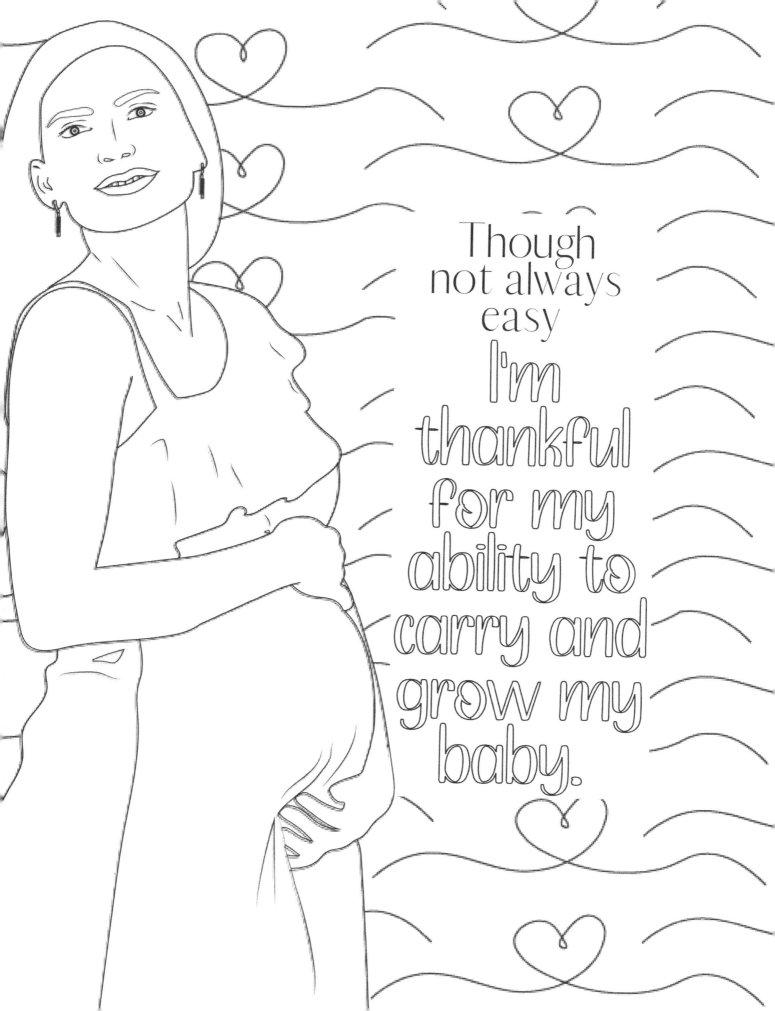

Though not always easy I'm thankful for my ability to carry and grow my baby.

I welcome the changes
in my
body
in my
life

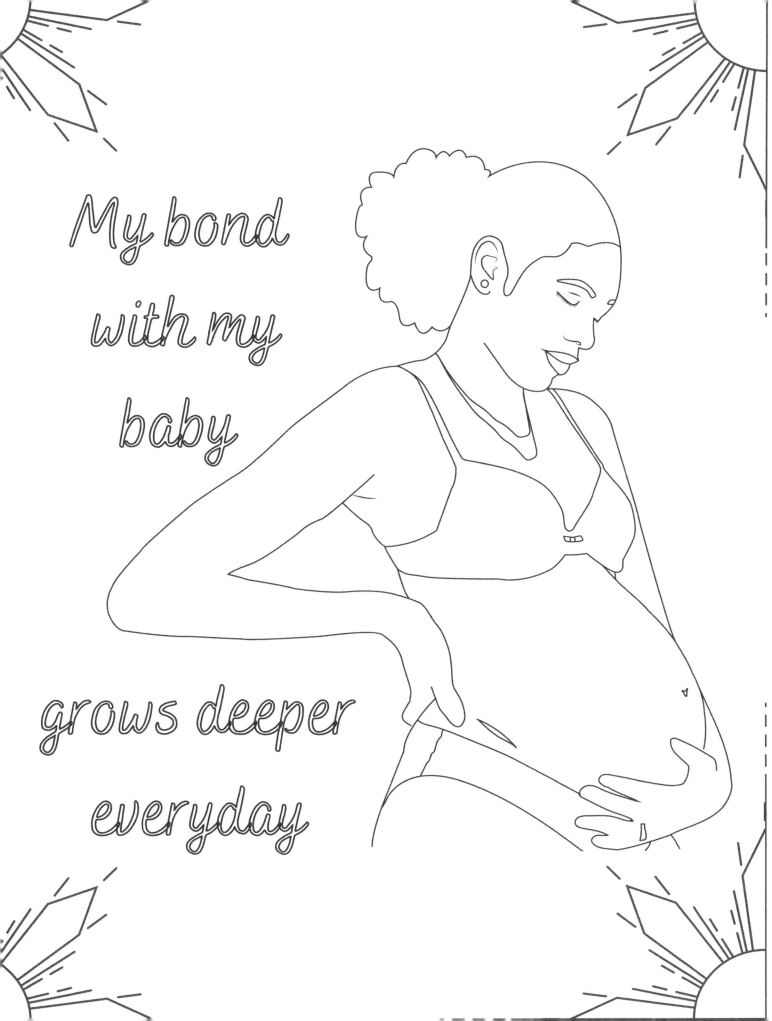

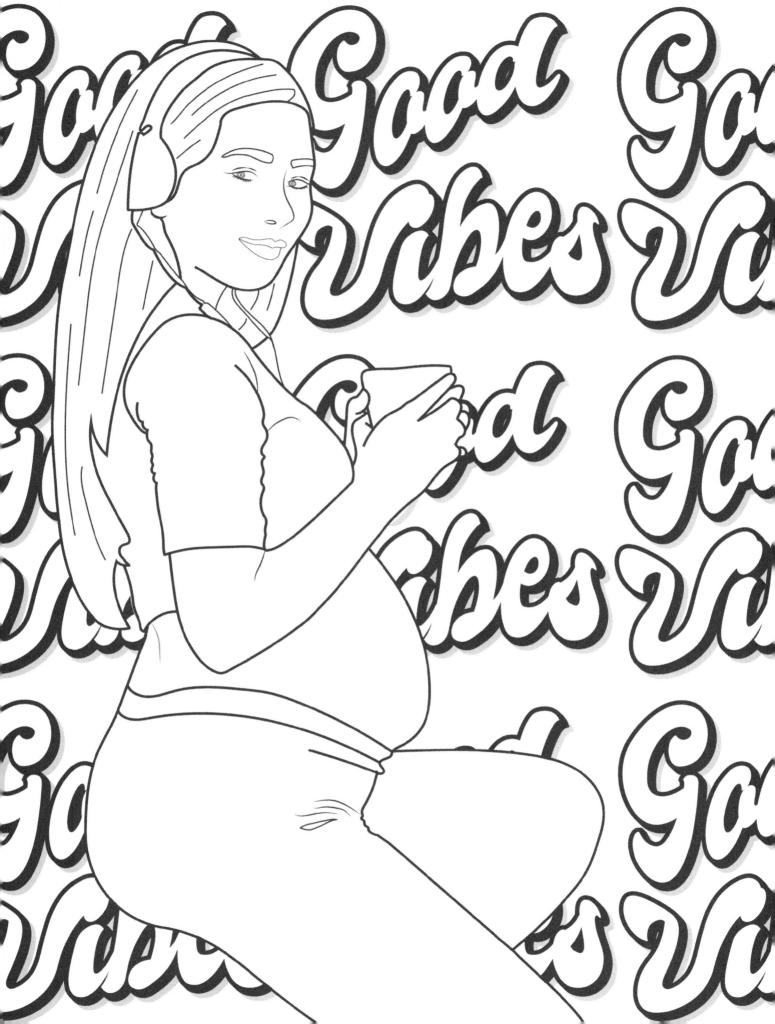

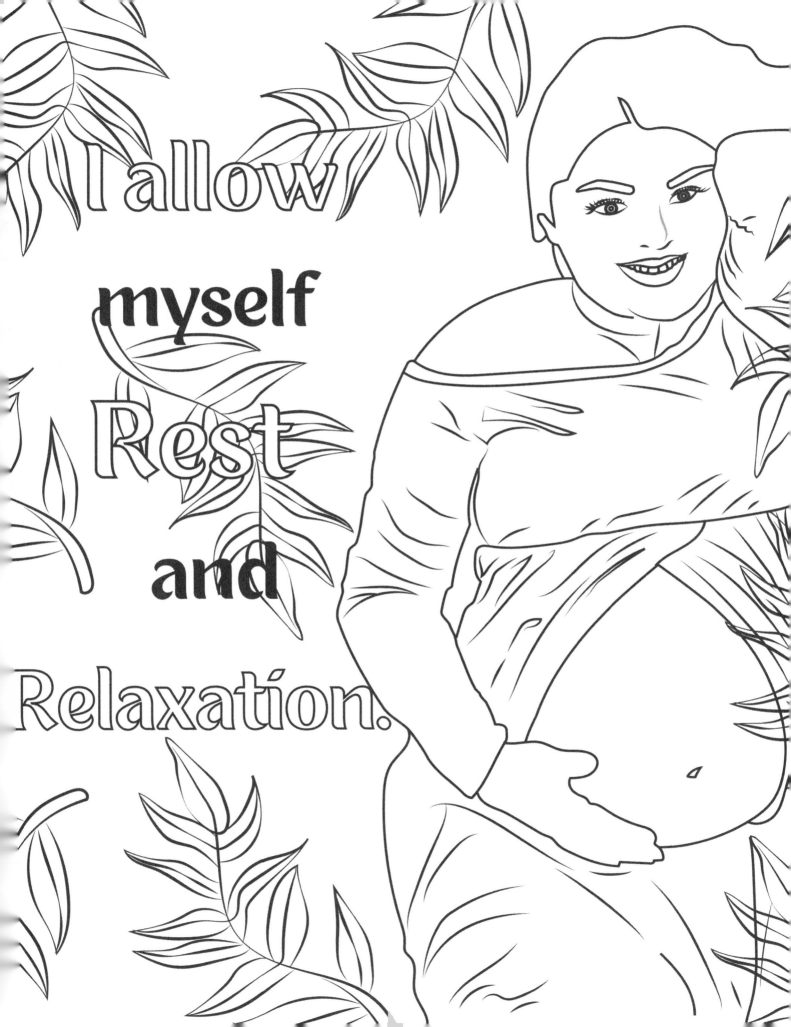

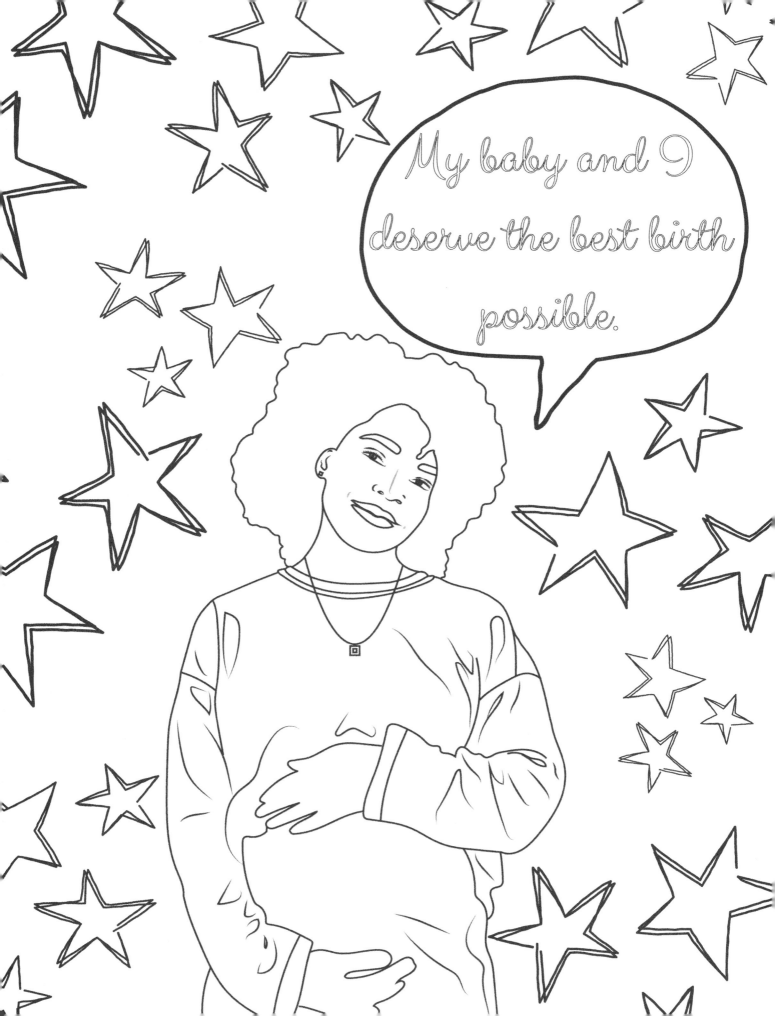

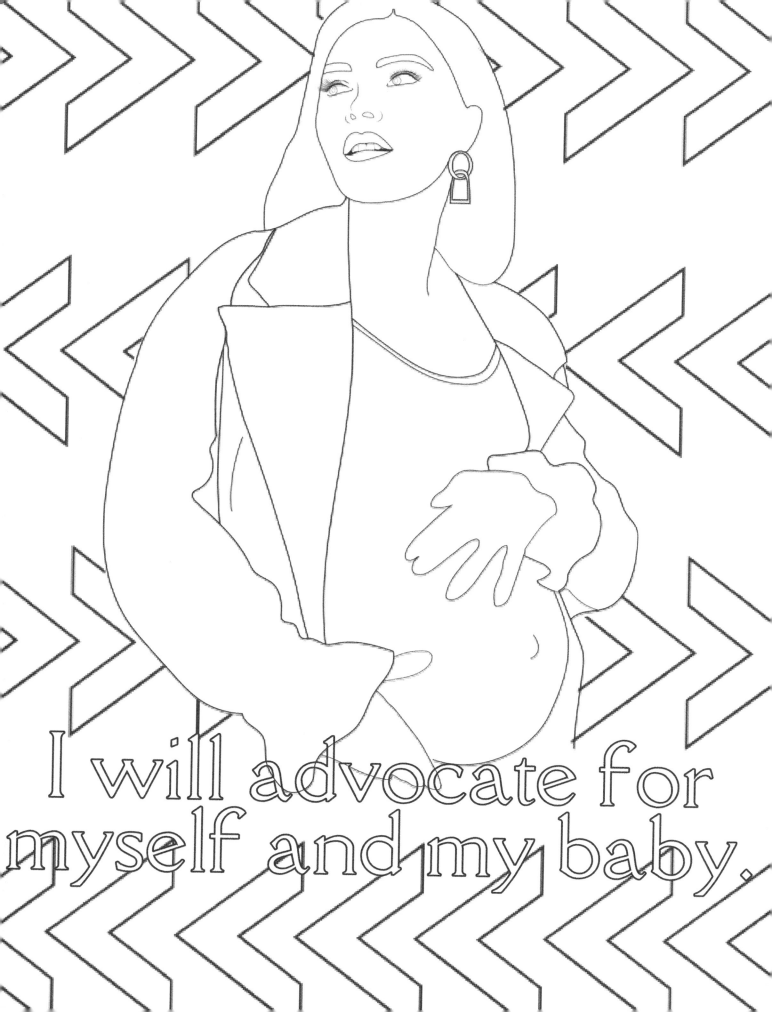

I take pride in my pregnant body... it is capable of amazing things.

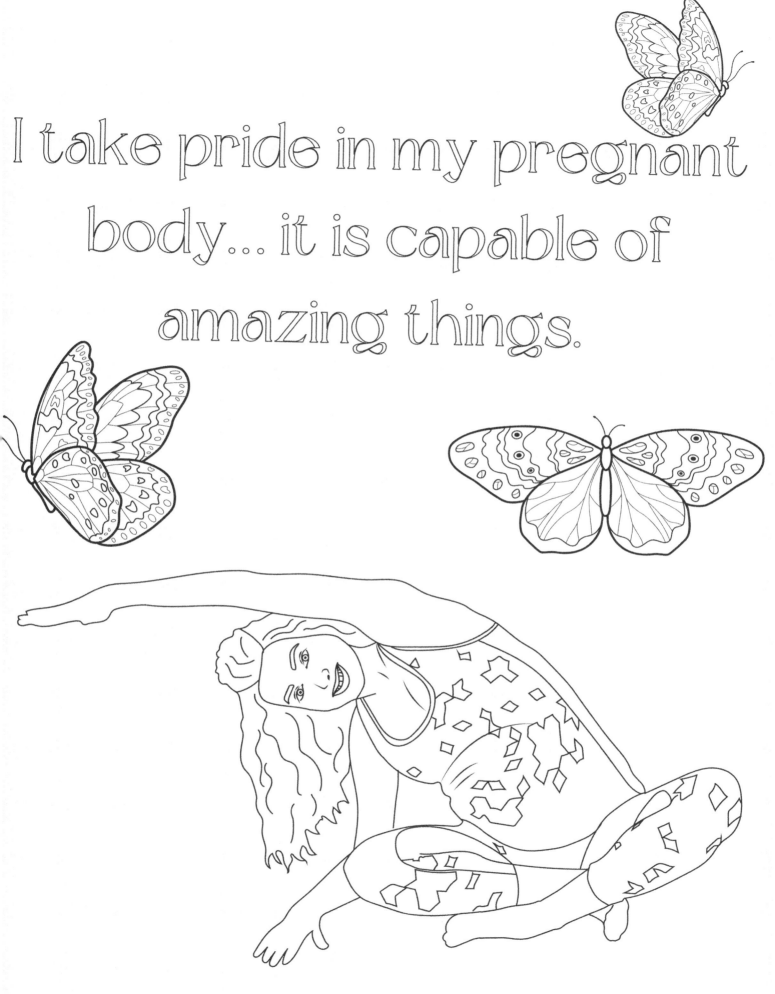

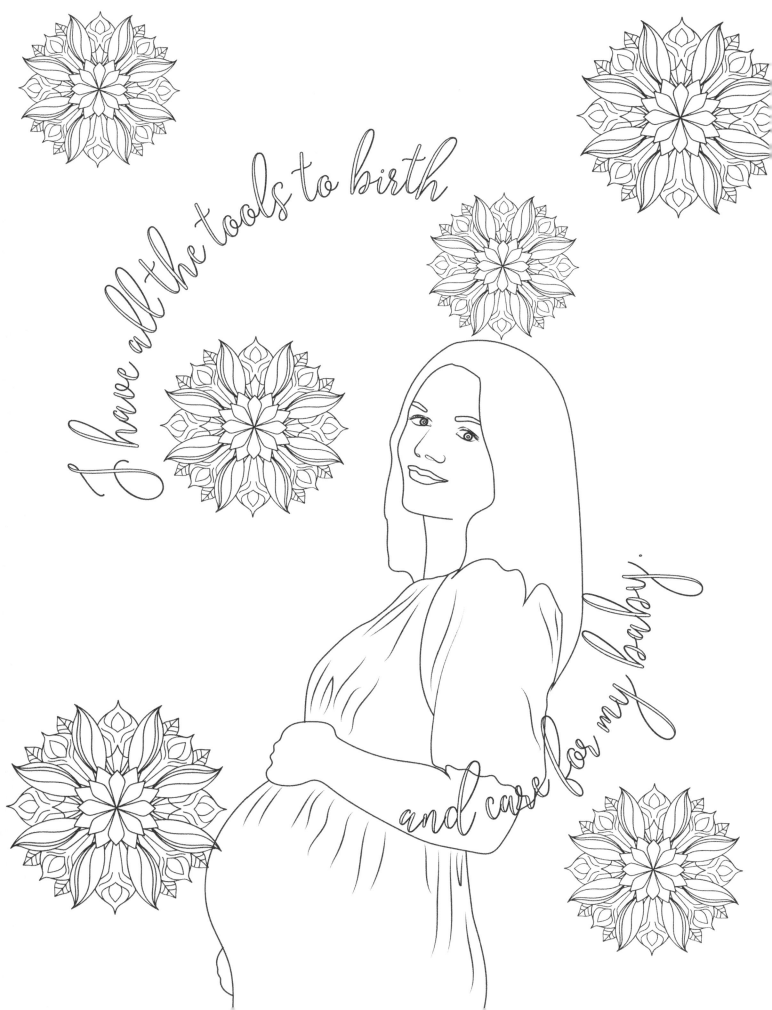

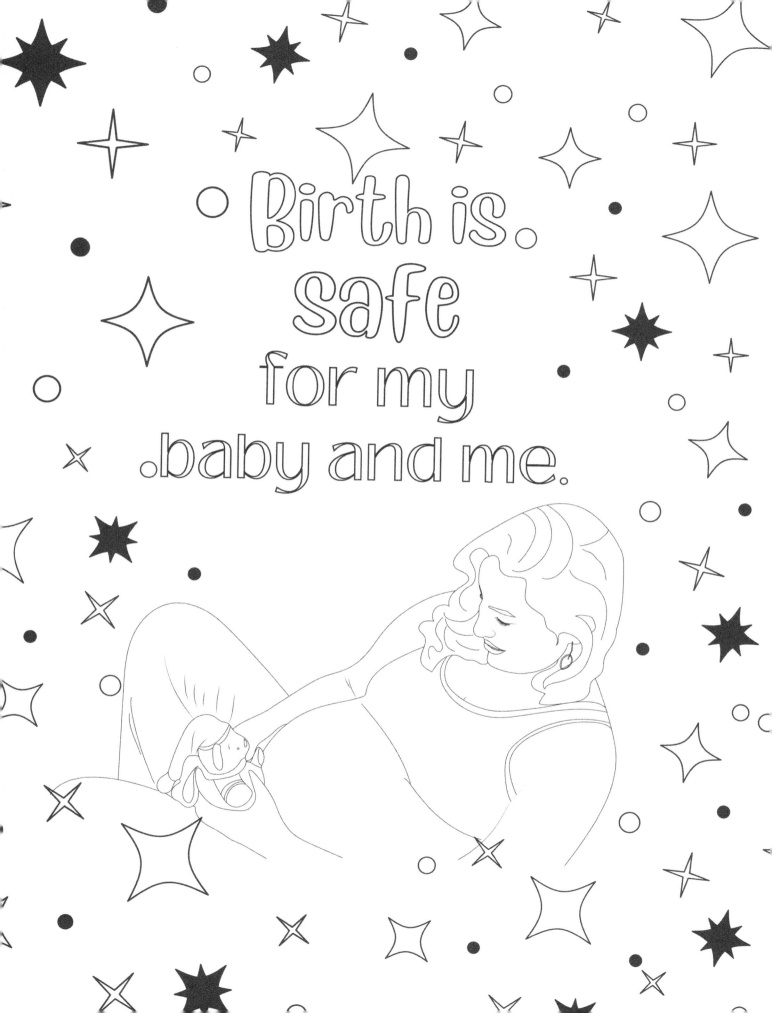

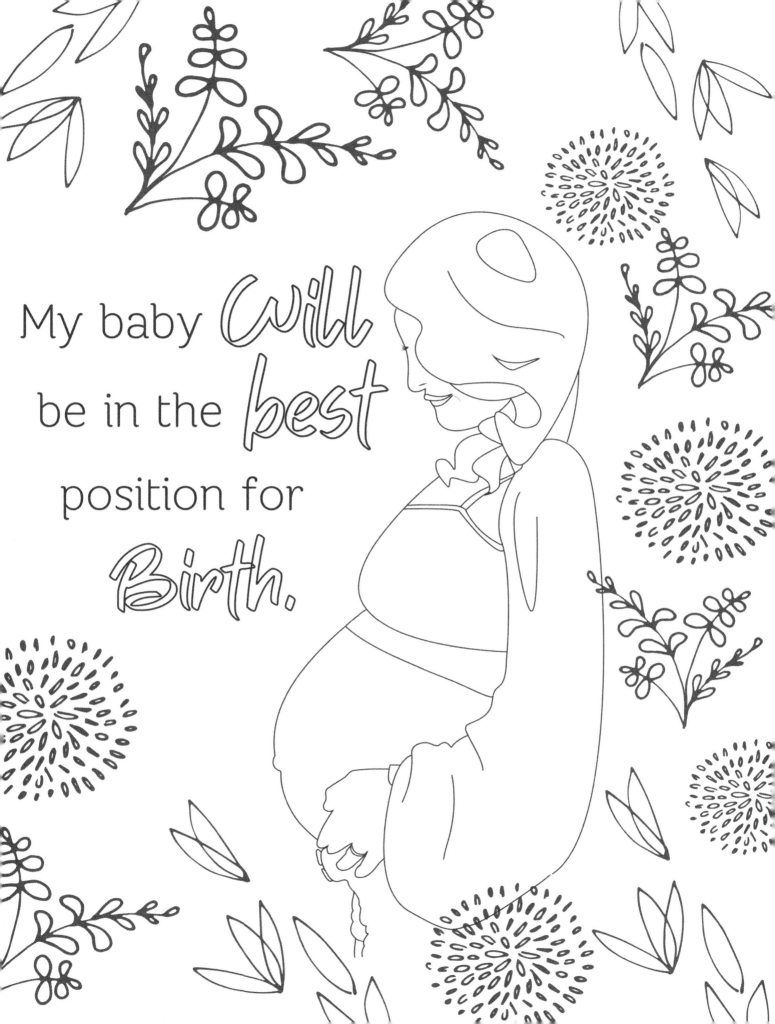

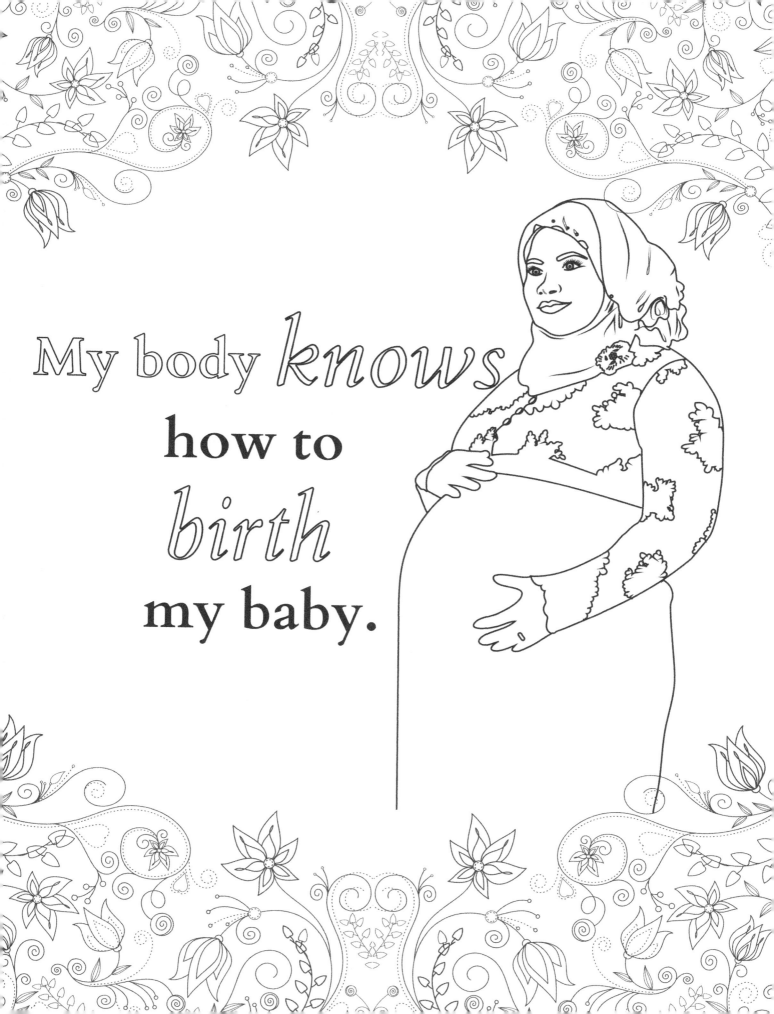

My body *knows* how to *birth* my baby.

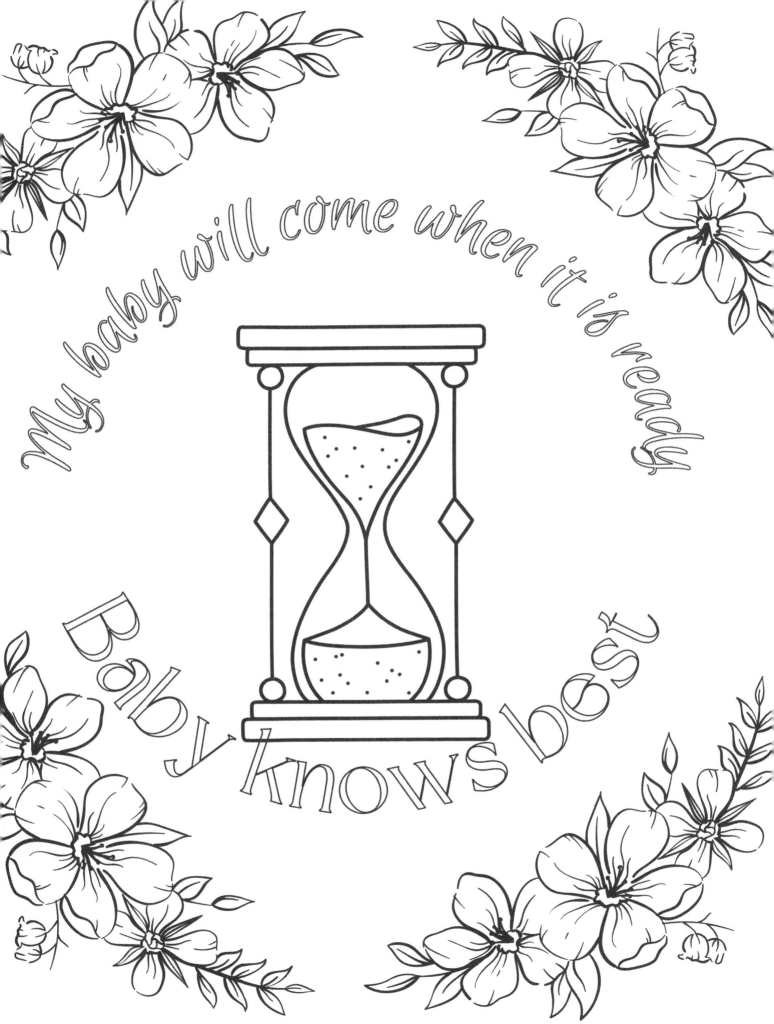

The Third
TRIMESTER

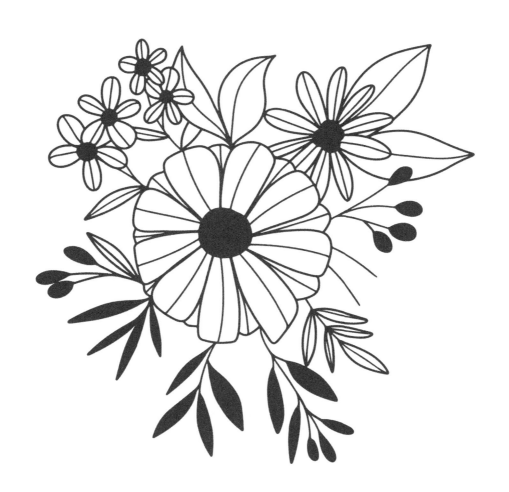

Amazing Momma

Growing a baby isn't easy. While some women will face different challenges than the next, we may all have moments of uncertainty, doubt, or even "what have I gotten myself into?"

In those moments know you are not alone. There is a community of women in this with you, there are resources dedicated to you, and most of all that your doing an amazing job being a mother (*even now*).

Though baby can't articulate their love or gratitude yet, please know it's growing as big as they are. In those challenging moments know your baby loves you and thanks you for all you are doing for them.

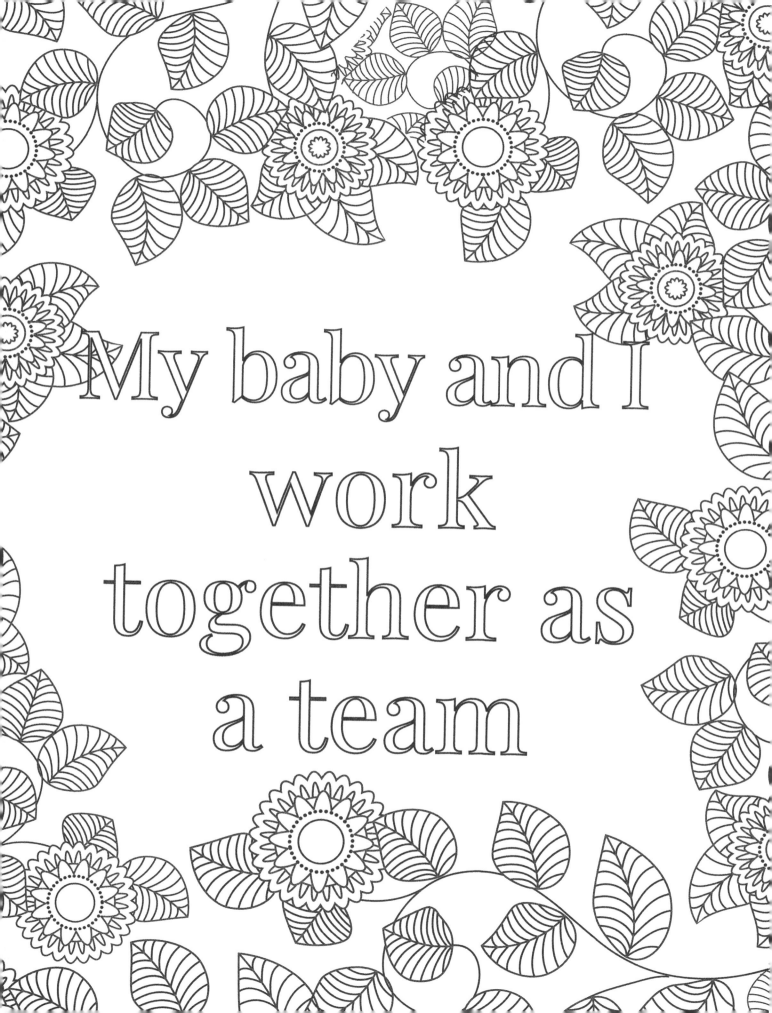

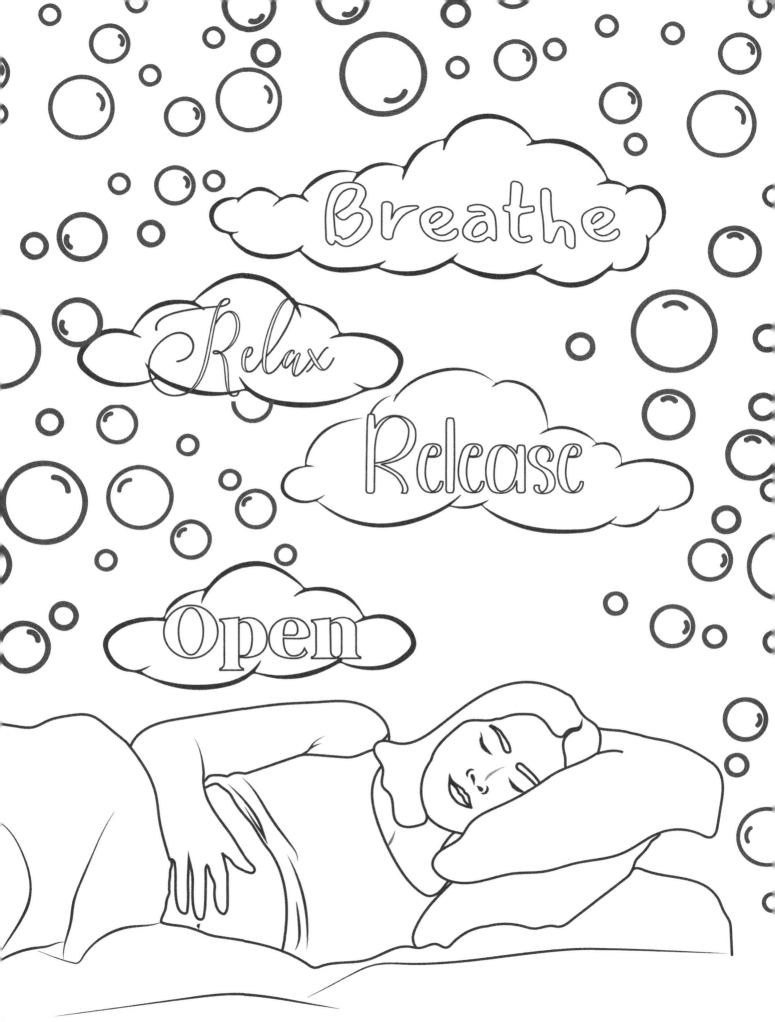

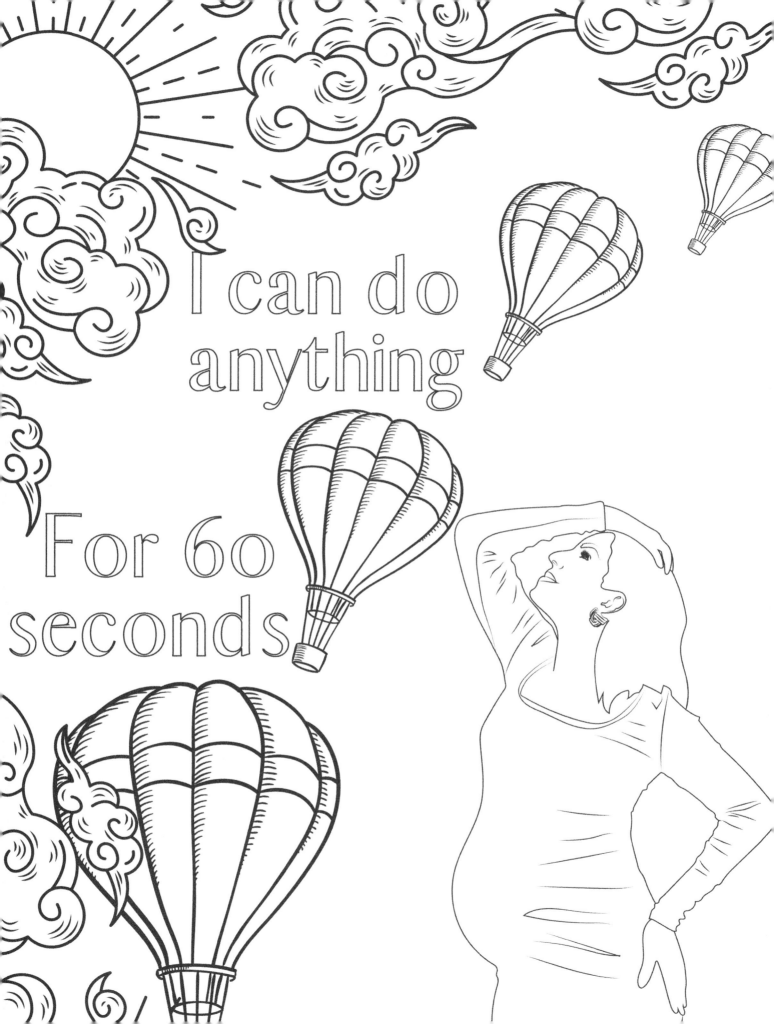

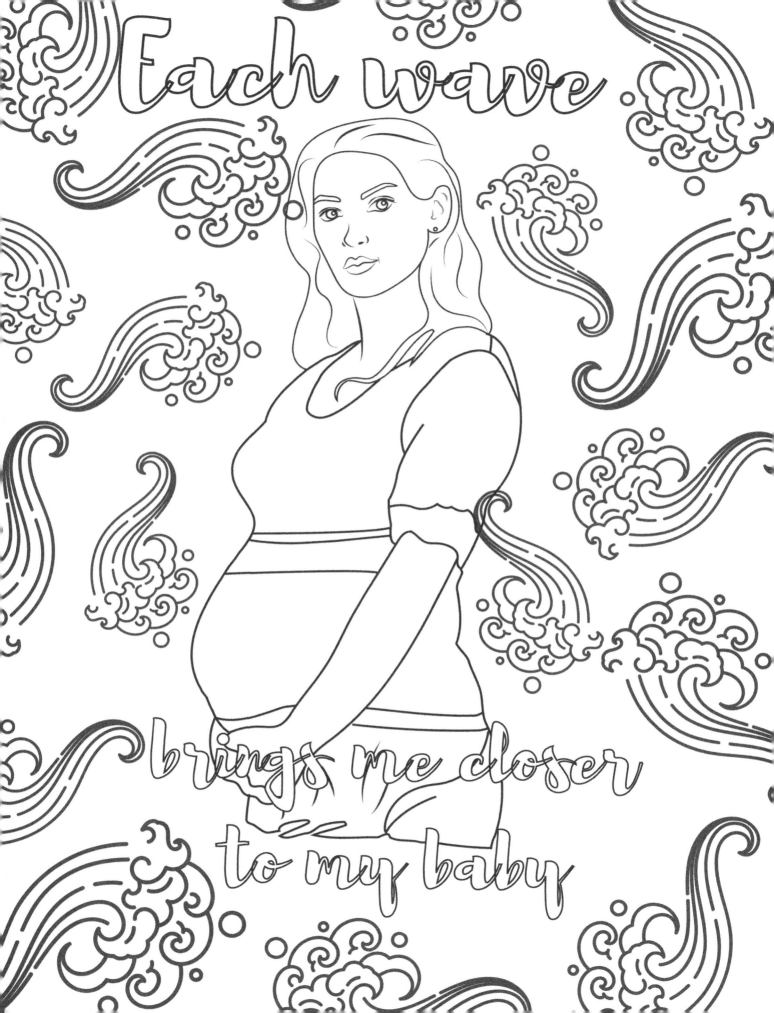

Breathe

BABY DOWN

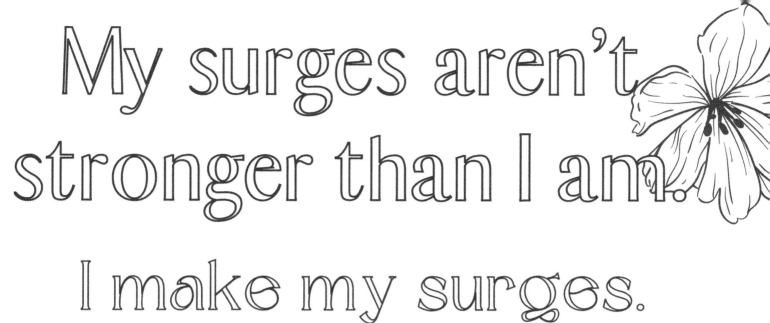

My surges aren't stronger than I am.

I make my surges.

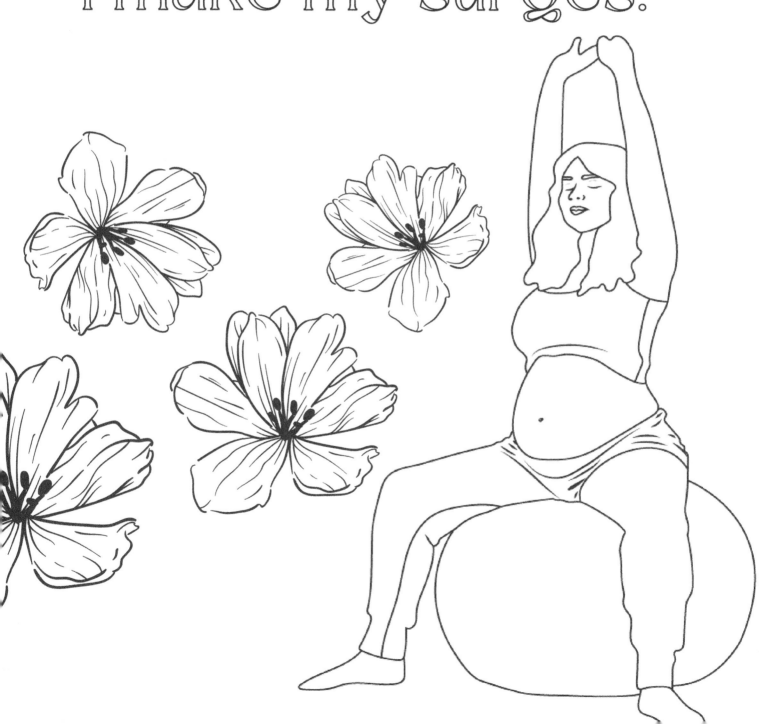

Women all over the world are laboring with me

I gain strength in knowing I'm not alone

I CAN DO THIS!

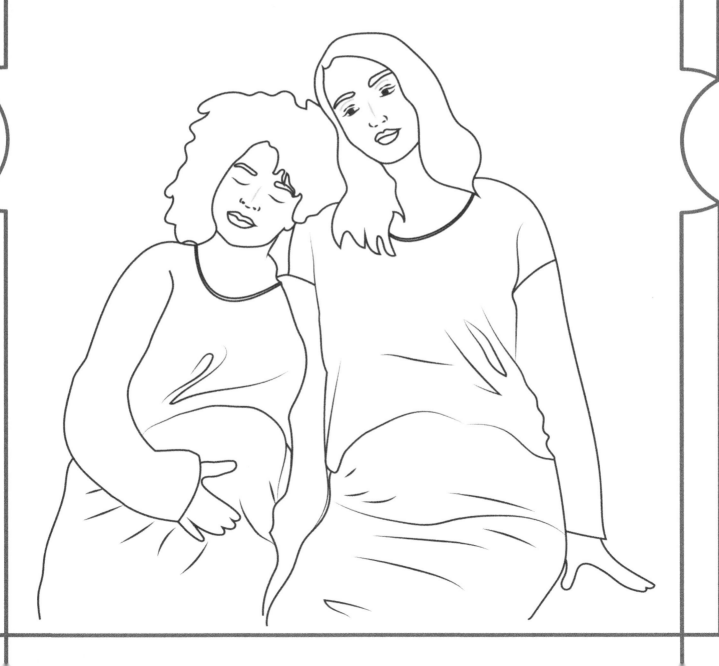

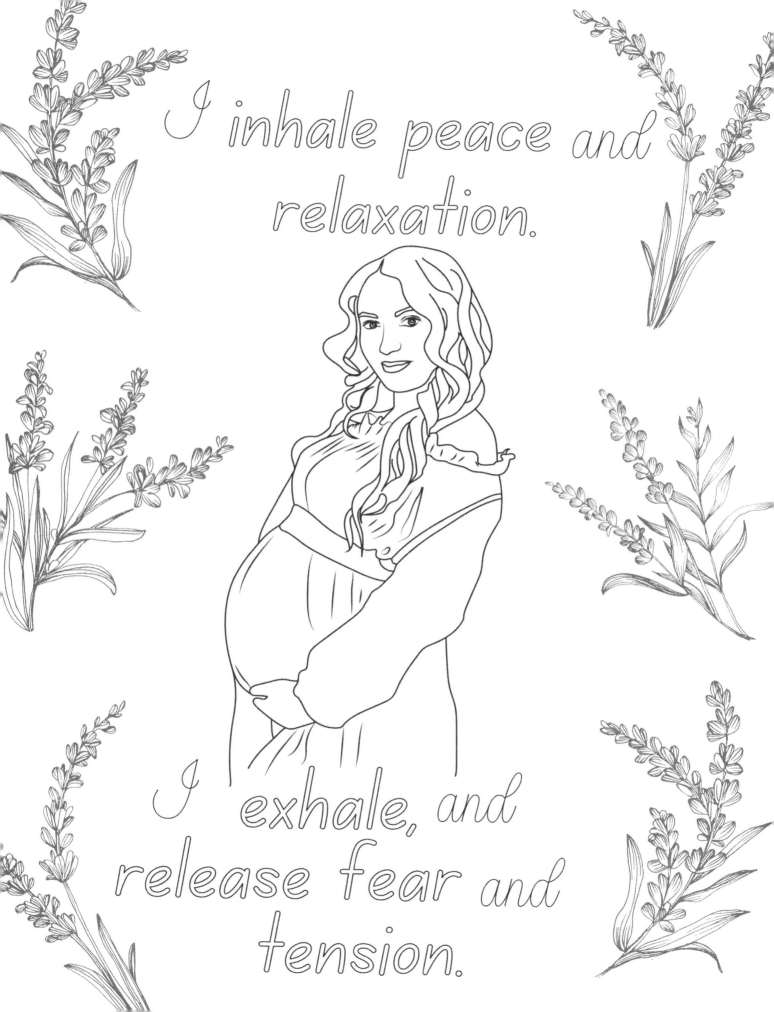

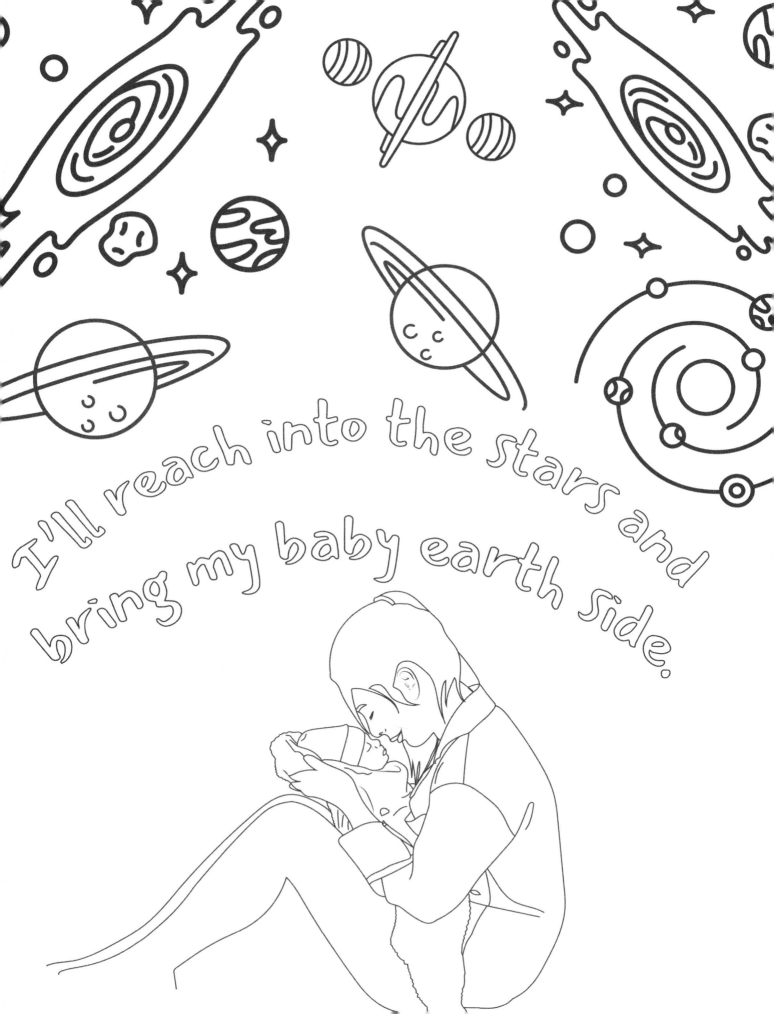

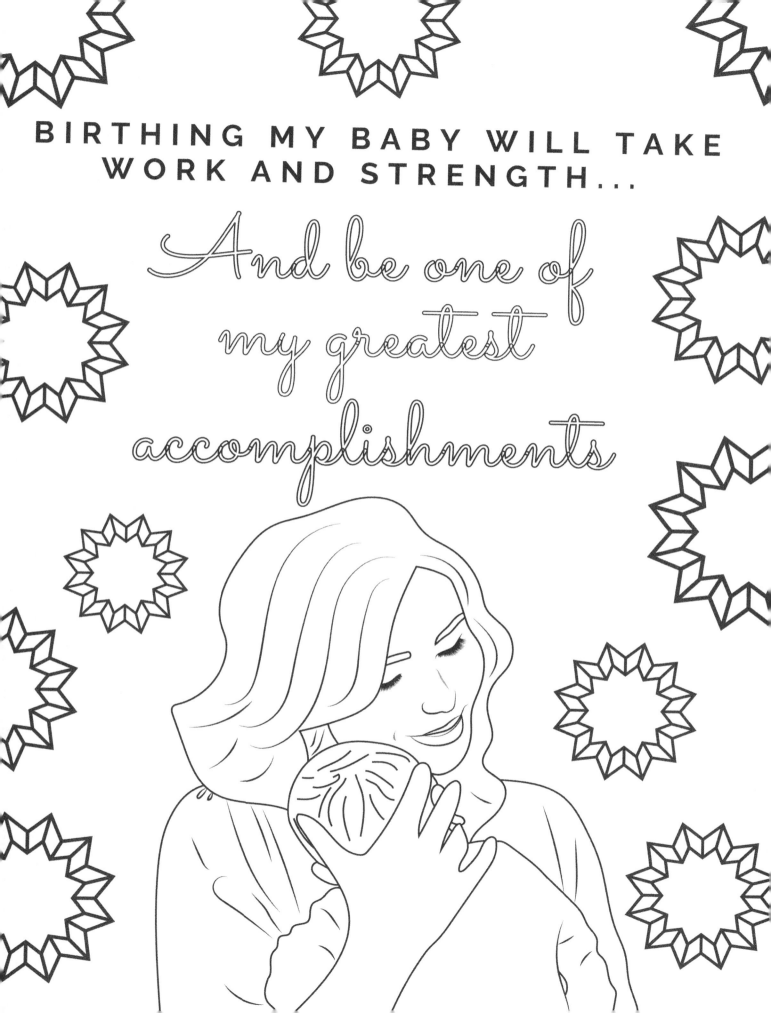

My baby and I will be

healthy & happy

strong   safe

after I give birth.

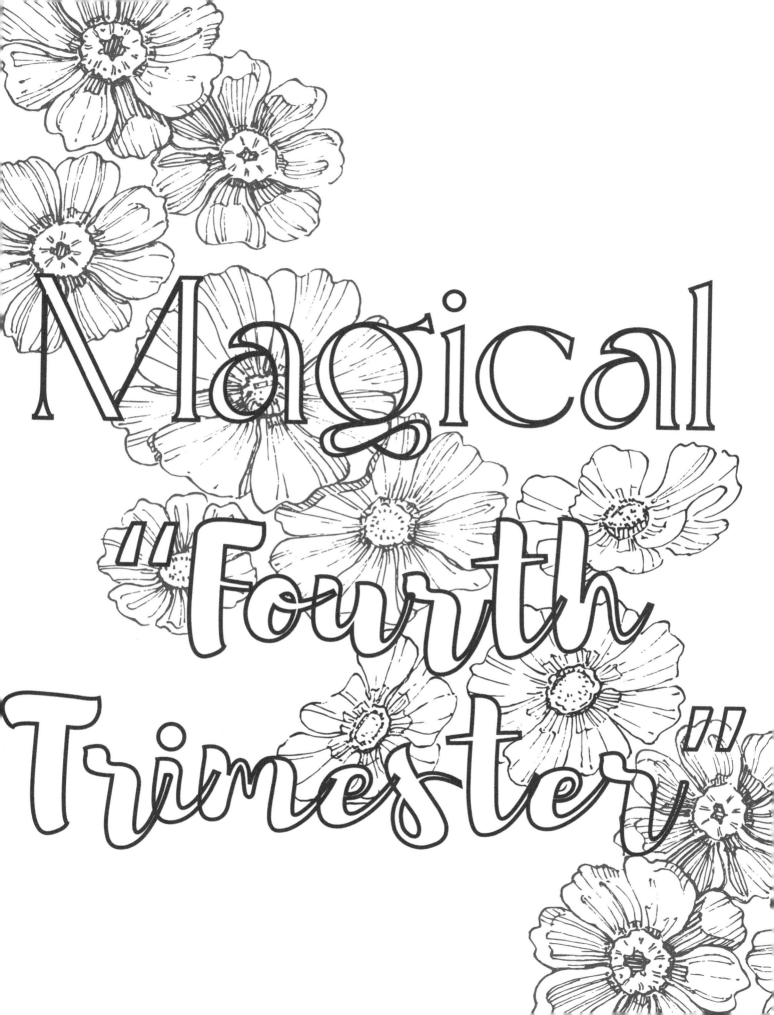

Incase no one told you

You've done it Momma! You've brought this amazing new life into the world! The hard part is over. Or is it?

So much energy and time is spent on the pregnancy, but the real adventure begins once you've given birth. Not only do you have a precious new soul to care for, but you may be balancing work, other children, a spouse/partner, or just life in general. At times you may feel pulled in many directions or even overwhelmed. In these moments remember those same resources and communities you discovered while pregnant are here for you now. You are not alone.

In these moments remember it is ok to carve out time for yourself and to nurture your own well-being as lovingly as you nurture your new baby. In these moments show that gorgeous postpartum body the respect it deserves. You just created and birthed a whole human. Whether you had a vaginal delivery or a c-section your body needs time to heal. So be kind to yourself and remember you are amazingly beautiful inside and out. Tell yourself this often because it can be easy to forget. Know without a shadow of a doubt you deserve happiness, care, and love too (in whatever way that looks like to you).

I can feed, care for, and nurture my baby.

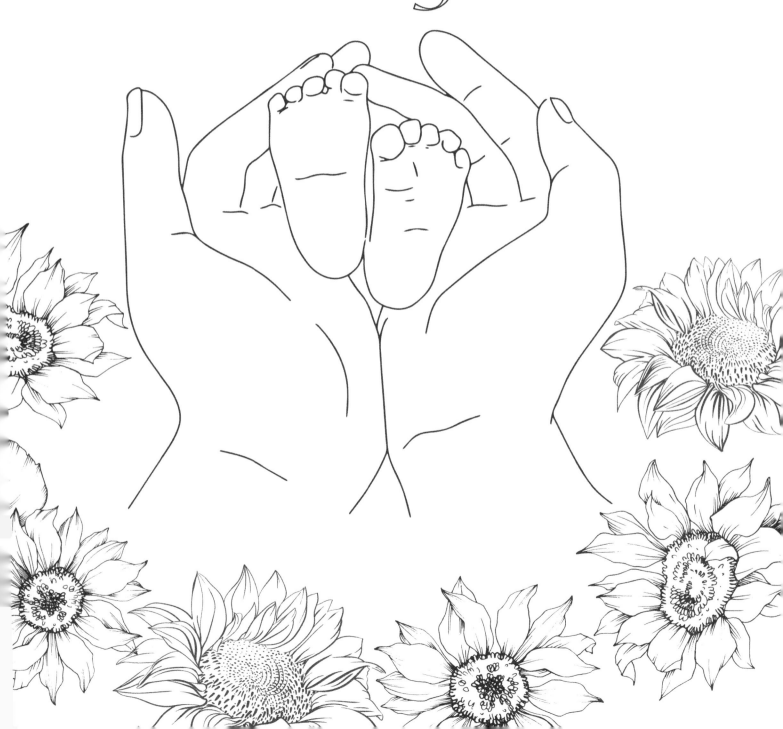

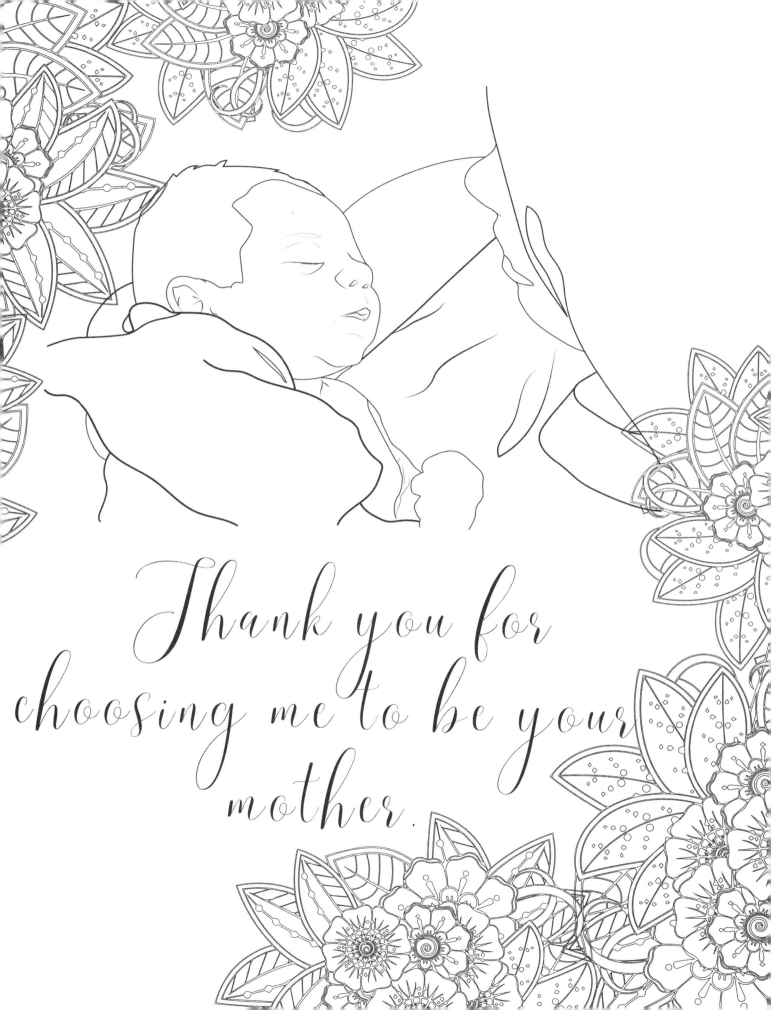

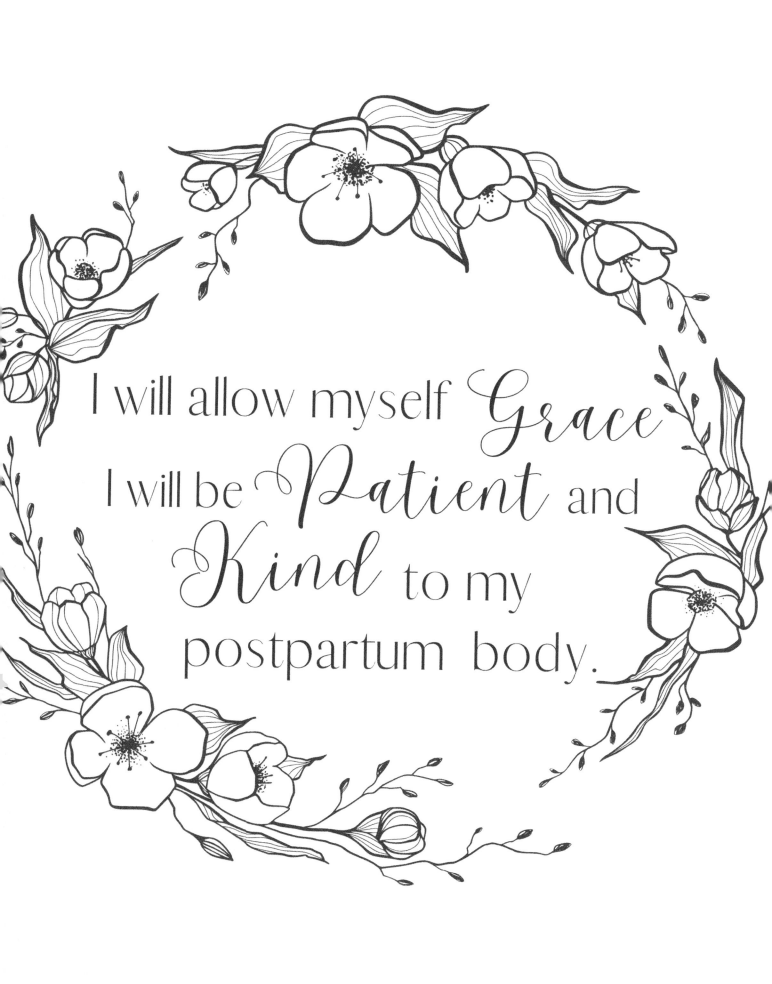

I will allow myself *Grace*
I will be *Patient* and
Kind to my
postpartum body.

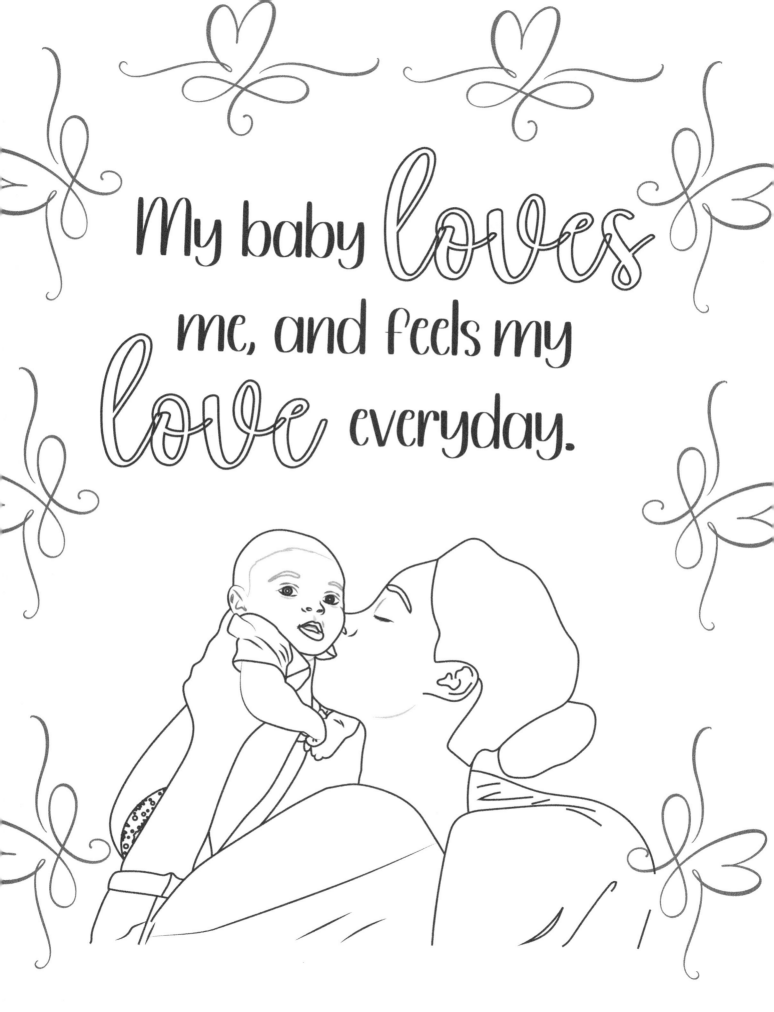

Though I'm imperfect

I AM THE PERFECT MOTHER FOR MY CHILD

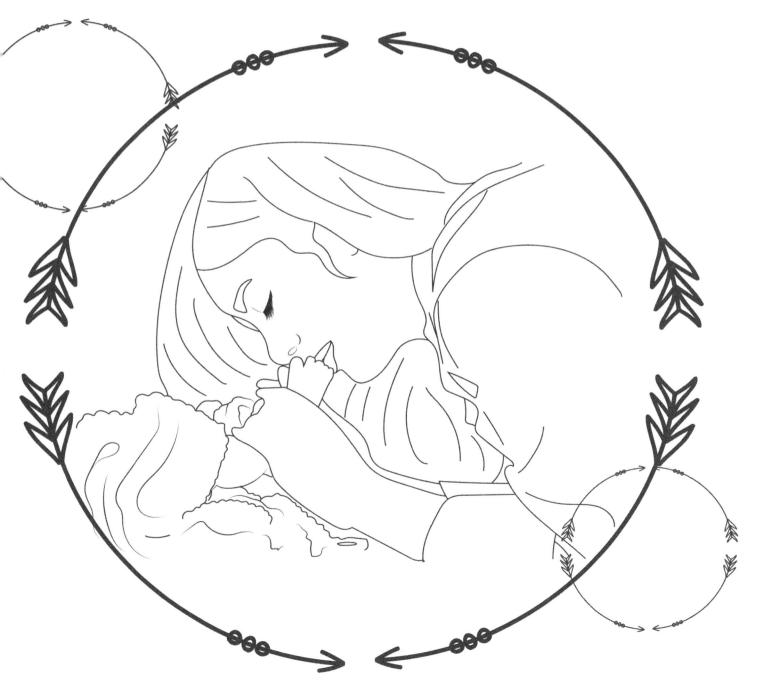

I will show myself love.

IN CARING FOR MYSELF I CAN BETTER CARE FOR MY FAMILY

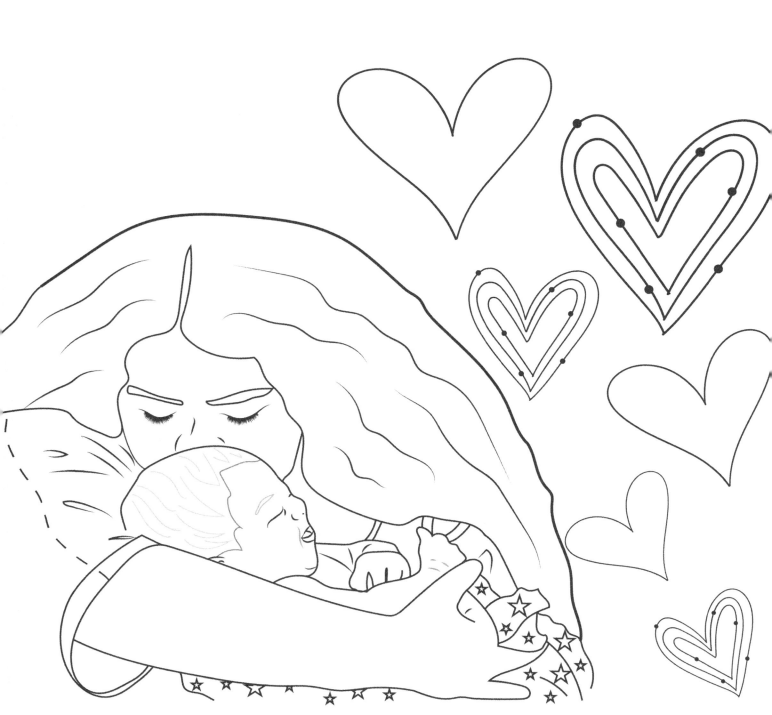

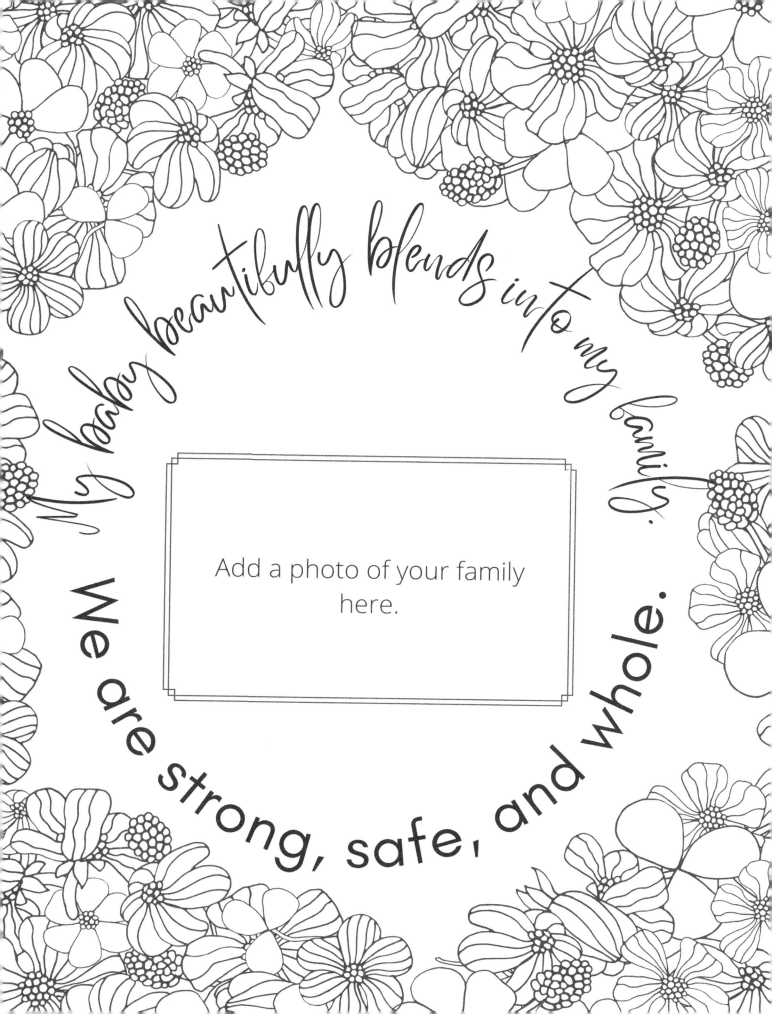

My baby beautifully blends into my family. We are strong, safe, and whole.

Add a photo of your family here.

thank you for your purchase

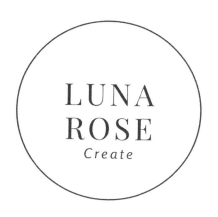

LUNA ROSE
Create

We hope you enjoy your order as much as we enjoyed making it. This is a true labor of love and to show our appreciation we at Luna Rose Create would like to offer you a Free Gift. Just visit the link below.

https://mindfulmomma.lunarose create.com/10pdfs

Reach out

Comments or concerns? Get in touch we are happy to help. Email us at

hello@lunarosecreate.com

If you are happy with your order please let us know and leave a review.

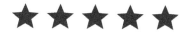

Made in the USA
Monee, IL
14 September 2022